Apple Cider Vinegar For Weight Loss

Simple Easy Solution For Quick Weight Loss and Increased Health

Dana Lee

<u>Published by:</u>

Dana Publishing
P.O. Box 1801, Mentor OH 44060
U.S.A.

<u>Legal & Disclaimer</u>

Upon using the contents and information contained in this book, you agree to hold harmless the Author from and against any damages, costs, and expenses, including any legal fees potentially resulting from the application of any of the information provided by this book. This disclaimer applies to any loss, damages or injury caused by the use and application, whether directly or indirectly, of any advice or information presented, whether for breach of contract, tort, negligence, personal injury, criminal intent, or under any other cause of action.

You agree to accept all risks of using the information presented inside this book.

You agree that by continuing to read this book, where appropriate and/or necessary, you shall consult a professional (including but not limited to your doctor, attorney, or financial advisor or such other advisor as needed) before using any of the suggested remedies, techniques, or information in this book.

Table of Contents

Introduction

"A Great Quick Resource For Learning About Apple Cider Vinegar and Its Health and Weight Loss Benefits/Potential!"

-    *Roger Goldsmith, Editor at InformationHacker.*

Apple Cider Vinegar Can Fast Track Your Weight Loss Naturally!

There hadn't been much research into the claim that APPLE CIDER VINEGAR helps with weight loss. However, once the obesity epidemic in the United States grew to the proportion it is now, people started to pay attention. It turns out that sipping on APPLE CIDER VINEGAR before a meal helps aid digestion, as you've already read, but it also controls what happens within your blood. It lowers blood sugar., and this can lead to weight loss. But it is a little more complex than just that.

In a recent study, those who drank a tablespoon of Apple Cider Vinegar mixed with eight ounces of water had lower glucose levels, helping them feel better, fuller, and make better, more responsible choices. "Acetic acid, the main component in vinegar, may interfere with the body's ability to digest starch," says lead study author Carol Johnston, PhD, associate director.

It is that starch-blocking ability that will help you lose that extra baggage, especially in your stomach and hips. "If you're interfering with the digestion of starch, less is being broken down into calories in the bloodstream. Over time, that might cause a subtle effect on weight," says Johnston. A few other studies back up the very same theory: Consuming two teaspoons of vinegar before eating a bagel and juice was shown to reduce blood sugar spikes in a 2009 Annals of Nutrition & Metabolism study, while Japanese research published that same year associated vinegar consumption with lower body weight, BMI, weight circumference, and serum triglycerides.

Don't expect miracles – you aren't going to lose twenty pounds in one week and isn't a free pass to eat plates and plates of Olive Garden pastas and breadsticks every night.

Chapter 1:
The History of Apple Cider Vinegar

Vinegar was likely a happy accident, created separately in different parts of the world; a bottle of wine or beer was too long uncovered, and a culinary legend was born. The legacy of vinegar dates back at least 8000 years; vessels with vinegar traces dating from 6000 B.C.E were found in Egypt and China.

It is reported that around 5,000 B.C.E. that the Babylonians used vinegar made with dates as a preservative and a condiment, and they started experimenting with aromatic kinds of vinegar using herbs and spices. While the usefulness of vinegar in the kitchen has been known for thousands of years, the first to prescribe vinegar for a range of diseases and preventive needs was Hippocrates (around 400 B.C.E.).

Hippocrates had long been known to use apple cider vinegar as a tonic for health. Since then, home remedy books and old maid's tales have all prescribed the treatment of this vinegar. Dr. Jarvis wrote a book in 1958 on the health benefits of apple cider. According to his instructions, cider vinegar should be mixed with sweet honey, and a teaspoon should be taken every day. By the 1970s, the popularity of apple cider vinegar had increased again. After reading his book, the proponents were used to create an apple cider vinegar weight loss plan.

Some remnants of apple cider vinegar found in a vase dating back to pre-Pharaonic times were found in Egypt, indicating that Egyptians were aware of it and used it to preserve food, just as the people of Babylon and Persia did. Vinegar can be used to carry food on long journeys. Mixed with water, farmers and travelers used it in ancient times to quench thirst.

Vinegar for disease and other health conditions has been used since the time of Hippocrates (roughly 460–377 B.C.). A Greek medical practitioner, known as the "father of medicine," used vinegar to purify injuries and to treat open and infected lacerations, and also prescribed a vinegar and honey combination for chronic respiratory conditions.

The "Mother" in Apple Cider Vinegar

Apple cider vinegar includes an all-powerful "mother," the sediment-like and cobweb-like material which can be seen in unfiltered ACV products. The mother contains concentrated bacteria and enzymes that make ACV so well known for its antifungal, antiviral, and anti-bacterial healing properties. Although some people can be put off ACV bottles by the water, this component is the product of special processing that preserves apple nutrients and enzymes during the fermentation process and thus offers specific curative powers for the ACV.

From Babylonians to Samurai Warriors

Vinegar is one of the oldest fermentation methods known to man, from Ancient Babylonians to samurai warriors. The earliest process of fermentation is wine from which the first vinegar had been made. The Babylonians, dated back to 5000 BC, made date palm wine, while the Egyptians made barley wine. Around 2500 BC, an ancient nomadic tribe called the Aryans made a sour wine from apples and this is considered to be a precursor for the cider. The word 'cider' is derived from the Phoenician 'Shekar,' which means wine or strong drink. So from the Babylonians, the Aryans, the Phoenicians, the Greeks, and the Romans got the soiled apple wine recipe, and people began to develop Apple cider vinegar as a byproduct of their soiled apple wines (Rose, 2006).

Apple cider vinegar has been used in medicine for thousands of years. It has been commonly used for a variety of conditions, including mushroom poisoning, dandruff, and toothache. During the American Civil War and World War I, it was used to treat battlefield wounds. Japanese warriors, the samurai, are thought to have drunk it to increase their strength and power. Ancient Persians drank the dilution of vinegar in apple cider to avoid the build-up of fatty tissue in the body while Romans used fire and vinegar in their Alpine conquest to break rocks. Vinegar has been used for food preservation for thousands of years and remains a valuable cleaning product today. In short, historical records indicate that apple cider vinegar from around the world is used in countless ways (Rose, 2006).

Ancient Greece

In Ancient Greece, Oxycrat was the most common beverage. water, vinegar, and honey were collected, mixed and preserved in individual vases (oxides). A remarkable physician, Hippocrates, whose doctrines ruled over Western civilization until the 18th century, (i.e., for more than 2,000 years) prescribed this mixture to treat wounds, sores, and diseases of the breath.

The Romans

The Romans drank "posca," a combination of water and vinegar that was sold on the streets in contemporary times. Posca was supposed to give you energy, while you would get drunk from wine. In Christian scriptures, it is said that the praetorian gave a sponge soaked in posca to Jesus on the cross.

It wasn't cruelty, but a symbol of the soldier's pity to a man on the cross. Acetabulum, a glass bowl used for serving vinegar, was always present at Roman banquets. Feasters would dip small pieces of bread into the vinegar and eat it throughout the meal to aid digestion.

Vinegar was contained in nearly all the recipes prepared by Apicius, a well-known Epicurean gastronomer in Roman times. Later, Columella, a Roman agricultural writer, left a few vinegar recipes; acid yeast has been used to favor fermentation, while incandescent bars and hot fir cones have been placed in wine to purify them.

The Romans had several vinegar sauces, ranging from very basic to the popular garum, which was the strange mix of ingredients to be combined with vinegar. The Romans invented the method of marinating fried fish. In his Naturalism History, Pliny the Elder recommends vinegar to treat various conditions and to make life more pleasant.

Vinegar was always available for Roman legionaries. Their daily meal before the battle was momentum, a salad made of garlic, onion, rue, goat milk, and coriander, coated with oil and vinegar.

Throughout military campaigns, vinegar was also used to quench thirst, and mixed with water, to purify the skin, to avoid and treat infections caused by camp life and small wounds.

Hannibal Barca, the famous Carthaginian general (247-183 B.C.), crossed the Alps with foot soldiers, knights, and elephants at the Piccolo San Bernardo Pass and so avoided the Roman-dominated sea during the decisive fight between Rome and Carthage. It's a famous event. It is less clear why he crossed the Alps. The paths are narrow and twisting, difficult for the massive elephants. Hannibal had huge branches between the rocks, which blocked the trail, setting them on fire. Then he had poured vinegar on hot stones, the stone was crumbly, and soldiers would smash them to get troops and animals through.

The Middle Ages and Beyond

Middle Ages

 The technique for the production of vinegar improved in the Middle Ages, and Agresto was first produced using green grapes that could counterbalance condiment fat, thanks to their freshness and slight acidity.

In 1394, the newly established Vinegar Producers Association in Orléans put manufacturing technology under a code of secrecy under the penalty of expulsion by its representative. This is why the Orléans vinegar is widespread, and the business is booming. By 1580 the town and its suburbs had 33 vinegar mills as local wine, which was not very acidic or fruity, was highly suitable for the production of vinegar.

The geographic position of Orléans was also favorable: it was the last maritime port for goods coming from the west. The ships traveling along the river were very slow because of the lack of water, and by the time the wine got to the port, it was ready for vinegar processing, by correctly mixing it with the local wine.

Vinegar and the Plague

The Black Death spread all over Europe and killed one out of three people in the 14th century. Until 1670, the outbreak of the disease was marked every year at different levels.

Vinegar was believed to be great for prevention, and the people of Marseilles shielded themselves from the "fever-creating" air in 1720, the year of the last major outbreak in western Europe. They kept a vinegar-swept sponge "under the nose" without ever breathing through the mouth or swallowing saliva. Nurses supported the doctors with a vinegar basin, in which the doctors could wash their hands before the patients palpated. When the force of the plague diminished, the walls of the homes where the sick lived were washed with vinegar.

Vinegar of the Four Thieves

In the novel 'Promessi Sposi' by Manzoni, a vinegar-treated bandage was placed around the foreheads of the Monatti- the carriers of the corpses- to avoid infections. Four of them (some people say 7) were able to sack the town scot-free during the 1720 plague outbreak in Marseille thanks to the ablutions and aromatic vinegar gargles of which the ingredients are unknown.

They were finally sentenced to death for sacking and robbery, but their lives were spared due to the vinegar they used, which became known as the Vinegar of The Four Thieves. The vinegar used in the four robberies was made by a French specialist, based on the original Marseilles recipe with many spices, cloves, and camphor and wormwood, and three pints of vinegar.

Vinegar and Cholera

A former infectious disease from remote regions of Asia, it is still prevalent in several countries in Europe and is often mistaken for acute gastroenteritis, with which it has a lot of similarities. Cholera has been treated with vinegar in any historical period. The government of Vienna passed an order almost two centuries ago (1830 and 1884), because of the cholera outbreak, that people had to wash their hands with vinegar before and after a visit to a friend or sick person, as well as fruit and vegetables before eating it. Cholera can be spread by water, so preventative action and the disinfection of food are well known.

Recent research by Franco Mecca (Franco Angeli Editore)

shows that vinegar has a "simple and marked" disinfectant effect on cholera and other intestinal pathogens. In between 30 seconds-2 minutes, the vibrios on the surface of fruit and vegetables in contact with vinegar are killed.

Vinegar as a Beauty Product

Kings and princes used vinegar in the last century as a beauty product. The king of Portugal, the queen of Holland, the queen of Belgium and the princess of Wales, were selected, as the ad published in "Il Secolo" on 15 February 1873 states, to announce "that [vinegar] gives water a pleasant fragrance and has tone and soothing qualities," prevents chilblains from developing and strengthens musculature. The same ads include ammonia vinegar salt used as a disinfectant to enter hospitals, lazar houses, and "other areas where dangerous exhalations occur." Vinegar was also used for cleaning purposes in ancient and modern times. As Misette Godard points out, the situation in the European cities at the time can only be understood by comparing it with contemporary Calcutta.

Vinegar, a Multi-Purpose Product

Vinegar is a multifunctional drug; women smelled vinegar in the 19th century to restore their senses if their corset was too tight or to cure headaches. The house lady would also leave a bottle of vinegar open next to a person with influenza to prevent sickness for those who visited him/her.

Our ancestors used vinegar in the manufacture of syrups, emulsions, salts, decoctions, mouthwash, sublimates, lotions, eyewash, soap, and buffers. Vinegar has also been used for rinsing, massaging, gargling, fomenting, shaving, washing, inhaling, showering, bandaging, plastering, and many other uses.

Chapter 2:
Apple Cider Vinegar for Weight Loss

Apple cider vinegar is a great aid in reducing excess body fats. Due to the acetic acid content of this miracle vinegar, your appetite is suppressed and you feel fuller easily. Furthermore, ACV interferes with your body's digestion of starch. As a result, your body absorbs fewer calories.

This transforms to reduced weight and lesser body fats.

In addition, ACV contains enzymes that helps boost your metabolism rate. Higher metabolism means more body fats burned. As a result, your body also retains less water, making you feel more energized. Also, ACV lowers blood sugar levels which translate to lesser insulin. Studies show that lower insulin level helps reduce body weight.

Along with healthier food choices and regular exercise, simply add 2 tablespoons of apple cider vinegar in 16 ounces of warm water mixed with 1 tablespoon honey and drink it every day. It is recommended to drink this mixture before each meal. You may also add 2 tablespoons of ACV on your tea with a tablespoon of honey or maple syrup. Remember; do not go beyond 2 tablespoons for every drink. Another tasty option is to add one to two tablespoons of Apple Cider Vinegar on your daily smoothie. This way, you are able to incorporate ACV in your diet without even realizing it.

Since apple cider vinegar is an all-natural product, it does not have any harmful side effects and you can take it for as long as you want. But of course, anything that is too much is harmful, so stick to 2 tablespoons per drinking session only. Also, the effect of apple cider vinegar on weight loss is not immediate and it varies depending on your body type. Some have lost 2 pounds in 3 weeks while others lost 4 pounds in a month.

For a more effective weight loss using apple cider vinegar, you can add banana to your diet as it contains potassium which lowers blood pressure. Banana is also known to reduce stress. Additionally, cut down your sugar intake as it can spike insulin levels. It will also help if you exercise more. For instance, you can have a 30-minute walk every day or go biking during weekends.

Chapter 3:
Natural Weight Loss using Apple Cider Vinegar:

Being overweight is embarrassing in addition to being uncomfortable. If you have been trying to lose weight and keep it off, you're probably ready to try something completely new.

Apple Cider Vinegar and Dieting:

ACV (apple cider vinegar) is a well-known natural remedy and is used by countless people to both cure and prevent common ailments. In addition, this liquid holds a crucial spot in the world of dieting. Scientific research along with personal experiences have proven that apple cider vinegar can, in fact, help you reach your ideal weight.

The Long-Term Answer:

Just treating the symptoms of a problem, without going deeper, will not provide a lasting solution. Apple cider vinegar is a substance that can target your weight problem from a holistic perspective, offering a long-term answer instead of a quick fix.

Proof and Research about ACV and Weight Loss:

This chapter is here to help you know how apple cider vinegar works, along with how you can use it day to day to improve your overall health and lose that extra weight.

One of the most interesting studies done on how this liquid can aid weight loss was done in the year 2009 by **Bioscience, Biotechnology, and Biochemistry.** This study found that drinking a couple of tablespoons of apple cider vinegar for a few months caused participants to lose significant amounts of body fat and waist circumference.

How Does Apple Cider Vinegar Help Your Body Shed Weight?

Apple cider vinegar comes from apples that are crushed, distilled, and finally fermented, as we went over earlier in the book. This results in acetic acid, a liquid that taps into some important physiological functions and supports the healthy loss of extra weight on your body. Let's look at some of the other reasons it helps you lose weight.

The Appetite Suppressant Effect:

Apple cider vinegar, first and foremost, helps you to eat less, causing your body to feel satisfied sooner than it normally would while eating. One study that showed this beyond doubt was done in 2005. The participants who ate their bread with some vinegar got full faster than the others who ate just bread.

The higher amount of acetic acid they consumed, the fuller the participants felt over the course of the study.

Blood Sugar Control for Weight Loss:

Apple cider vinegar helps to control your levels of blood sugar, as mentioned previously. It prevents those uncontrollable spikes in sugar and the crashes that lead you to want to snack in between the main meals of the day.

Once your blood sugar levels are stable, you will find it easier to eat just when you're hungry and stay with your diet. The study mentioned before also kept track of blood sugar levels with both the control group and vinegar group.

Study participants who consumed apple cider vinegar had much lower blood glucose levels after their meal. In other words, there wasn't the spike that usually comes after a high-carb meal. In addition, the ones who consumed larger doses of apple cider vinegar were still benefiting from the impact an hour and a half after they ate.

It helps to Prevent the Accumulation of Fat:

Apple cider vinegar helps to stimulate your body's metabolism function which helps you burn more fat faster. In addition, it has a lot of enzyme and organic acids that help you burn more fat by speeding your metabolism up.

Insulin Secretion and Apple Cider Vinegar:

Did you know that insulin plays a role in your body's storage of fat? It's true. Insulin is closely related to your levels of blood sugar, and the secretion of this hormone is disrupted in those who suffer from diabetes (type 2).

Some scientists suggested that apple cider vinegar could work very similarly to diabetic drugs, controlling this disease. For helping to cure your diabetes, diet is highly important. Do plenty of research into the foods and spices you should be consuming.

Apple Cider Vinegar's Detoxing Effect and Weight Loss:

When your body sheds harmful toxins, metabolism and digestion become much more efficient than before. Apple cider vinegar flushes out your body, allowing it to make the best use of the nutrients you eat. It also has high levels of insoluble fiber, improving bowel movements and absorbing toxins.

Which Type of Apple Cider Vinegar to Use for Losing Weight:

We've gone over this for other health benefits of apple cider vinegar, but it's especially crucial for weight loss. When you are using the liquid for this specific purpose, it must be raw and unprocessed. Better yet, use the kind you are making at home.

You should know by now that you should only be using apple cider vinegar that still has the mother intact to get the best benefits possible.

Avoiding Pesticides:

Apples are one of the most heavily sprayed fruits out there, when it comes to pesticides, making organic choices very important! You must purchase unfiltered, unprocessed, raw apple cider vinegar to get the benefits you seek and to lose weight, or just make your own.

Brand isn't as Important as Other Factors:

You may be wondering which brand of apple cider vinegar to use for weight loss, but brand doesn't matter as much as some other considerations. Any apple cider vinegar brand that is organic, unfiltered, and unpasteurized may be used for this reason.

One very common brand of organic apple cider vinegar is Bragg. You can buy this on the Internet, in health food stores, or in ordinary supermarkets, sometimes.

Don't worry about the apple cider vinegar not being pasteurized, since vinegar has a high enough level of acidity to kill off E. Coli and other harmful bacteria. Keep in mind that many doctors say that pregnant women shouldn't consume unpasteurized foods.

Steps for Using ACV to Lose Weight:

For those who don't like or are not accustomed to the flavor and impact of apple cider vinegar, you can start by including the liquid gradually in your diet, being careful not to use too much. This will prevent adverse effects.

<ins>How to Start:</ins>

You can begin by adding just a teaspoon of the vinegar to a glass of water, drinking this mixture at least one time per day. You can slowly increase the amount every time and how often you drink it.

<ins>The Optimal Amount to Drink:</ins>

According to studies on apple cider vinegar and weight loss, the ideal amount to consume per day is two tablespoons, diluted in water. Dilution is important because the liquid is highly acidic and dilution helps to protect your stomach lining, throat, and teeth.

<ins>Using a Straw:</ins>

Don't ever drink apple cider vinegar undiluted, this will cause you more harm than anything else. You may drink the diluted mix of apple cider vinegar and water using a straw. This will keep your tooth enamel safe.

<ins>Using Honey with Apple Cider Vinegar:</ins>

Some people will discover that the apple cider vinegar taste is hard to stand. In order to make the flavor more tolerable, you may add a little honey to it. The honey will mix better if you use warm water.

Mixing apple cider vinegar and honey have benefits for your health, and it also tastes great. If you are aiming to lose weight, try not to use too much honey as sugar can get in the way of weight loss.

Adding Apple Cider Vinegar to Food:

Soups: Apple cider vinegar can be used with certain foods and goes especially well with meat or bean soups. Just keep in mind that you should add the vinegar to your food after it has cooled. This will prevent the loss of nutrients to the heat. **Salads**: Apple cider vinegar is a popular dressing for salads and tastes especially great with olive oil and herbs added.

Pickling: For those who enjoy pickles or similar flavors, you can use apple cider vinegar to pickle cucumbers or other vegetables.

Herbal Tea: For those who don't mind the taste of apple cider vinegar, you can add it to your herbal teas to get the health benefits. This book will go over some other recipes later on.

How Often Should You Drink it?

In order to jump-start your metabolism and get the benefits of feeling full, some say that you must drink diluted apple cider vinegar an hour before eating to help you lose weight and improve digestion.

Morning Vinegar:

Some swear by drinking their apple cider vinegar right when they wake up and have empty stomachs. But others prefer not to do this. If you aren't comfortable drinking it without food in your stomach, you can do it after meals.

After Meals:

If you're more comfortable consuming apple cider vinegar after meals, you can do this two to three times per day. If you feel nausea or burning in your stomach, reduce how much you're taking.

Taking Breaks:

Some people recommend not consuming apple cider vinegar every single day and making sure to take breaks every month or so. As you can see, it all depends on what suits you best.

Possible Side Effects of Apple Cider Vinegar:

ACV is considered generally safe for human consumption, but as with all traditional remedies, you should take some precautions to make sure you're safe. Too much apple cider vinegar could lead to lowered levels of potassium in the body, causing osteoporosis.

But this effect happened to someone who drank 8 oz. of ACV every day for multiple years in a row. As you can see, we recommend jutting a couple tablespoons diluted every day, which is more than safe to consume regularly.

As said before, acidic items like apple cider vinegar can lead to weaker tooth enamel, so to prevent that, just rinse the mouth out with water each time you drink the apple cider vinegar mixture. Use a straw, too, to prevent tooth problems. You might also wish to refrain from brushing your teeth right after taking your apple cider vinegar mix.

Asking your Doctor about Interactions:

Apple cider vinegar may interact with diabetes medications, heart medications, laxatives, or diuretics. If you're on any meds, make sure you ask your physician before you decide to drink apple cider vinegar regularly.

Why is Apple Cider Vinegar Superior to Other Types for Losing Weight?

Apple cider vinegar is believed to be the best choice when it comes to weight loss, due to all of the health advantages it offers. It will clean your body, offering anti-microbial effects.

Considering the fact that it can aid high blood pressure, heart issues, diabetes, digestion, acid reflux, and possibly even kidney stones, it's obvious why apple cider vinegar is the best type of vinegar to use for health reasons.

What Should You Expect Using Apple Cider Vinegar To Lose Weight?

Apple cider vinegar should not be expected to give you an instant cure for a weight problem. The changes you see will happen on a gradual basis, but they will be permanent.

Patience is Key:

Remember to be patient, letting it work. At times, losing a pound per month and keeping it off is the real path to success. Don't get impatient and give up!

Other Factors in Weight Loss:

Also, keep in mind that the rate at which you lose your weight does depend on your other lifestyle habits, like genetics, stress, nutrition, and how much you exercise.

Making the Apple Cider Vinegar Work Better and Faster:

To get the fastest and best results, you have to combine this remedy with other proven methods. That way, the apple cider vinegar will work along with these other changes and give you the results you're hoping for.

Avoid Processed Foods:

If you're hoping to lose weight, you must avoid processed foods, unhealthy fats, and sugar. All of these will counteract the effects of the vinegar.

Find some Exercise You Enjoy:

Even moving moderately up to five times each week can help you speed up your metabolism and lose weight faster. Start by walking for 10 minutes each day and work your way up.

Potassium-Rich Foods:

If you eat foods that have plenty of potassium, this mineral can lower your blood pressure and reduce your stress levels. Spinach, avocados, sweet potatoes and bananas all have high amounts of potassium.

Chapter 4:
Other Uses of Apple Cider Vinegar

Acetic acid is the element that resides in vinegar and gives it its scent and taste. It also has effects on the body health.

One folk medicine used to **aid people with diabetes is this vinegar**. Several experiments have shown that before going to bed, drinking apple cider vinegar would give much more beneficial levels of blood sugar in the night. It also helps boost the amount of good cholesterol and lower the amount of fat in the body.

You can also use apple cider vinegar to help give **relief when you suffer from dandruff.** You help restore the acidic equilibrium on your scalp by mixing the vinegar with water and applying the solution to your hair. This approach is usually used for fifteen minutes at a time, only once or twice a week.

You can also use apple cider vinegar **to help cure acne**. This treatment is along the same lines as the cure for dandruff. Vinegar is mixed with water and dabbed into your skin's affected areas. But, be wary of this one. If the solution has too much vinegar, the vinegar will burn the body.

If you choose to use vinegar in your home remedies, you should be careful. You risk damaging your throat and teeth if you drink vinegar. You should consult your doctor before using vinegar in your diet if you have low potassium levels or osteoporosis. If you use too much, you may also damage your stomach and liver.

If you are still searching for more information about the

advantages and drawbacks of using apple cider vinegar, a quick online search will help you find out more, or pick up one of our other two books on ACV (See end of this book). There are plenty of resources out there to tell you what remedies you should look for and use. It's up to you!

It is sold in liquid form that is not filtered and unpasteurized. The mother of vinegar is found deposited at the base of the water in deep soil containing primarily acetic acid. Unlike others used to bake, this vinegar is used for health purposes. It is confirmed that diseases such as indigestion and pneumonia have been controlled. Several individuals have been treated by the use of apple cider vinegar combined with honey for digestive tract infections caused by bacteria.

Some studies have shown that lowering blood glucose levels can help people with diabetes.

Health Benefits

Proponents argue that apple cider vinegar (and vinegar in general) can improve your health in a variety of ways. A few of these claims are supported by science. Here's a glance forward.

Blood Sugar Level

The acetic acid in vinegar appears to obstruct enzymes that help absorb starch, leading to a smaller sized reaction of blood glucose after starchy meals like pasta or bread.

Scientists examined previously published medical research studies on the effects of vinegar intake with a meal in a report released in 2017 and discovered that vinegar assisted in reducing blood sugar and insulin levels after a meal.

Attempt adding a splash to salads, vinaigrettes, sauces, and marinades to integrate apple cider vinegar into your meals. If you have prediabetes or diabetes, make sure to talk to your doctor if you are thinking about using more substantial quantities that are generally used in baking.

Vinegar can interfere with treatment for diabetes, and people with certain forms of nutritional conditions, such as gastroparesis, should not use it.

Acne

Acne forms a plug (a blackhead or a whitehead) when keratin, the main protein in your skin, builds up in a pore. Unlike citric acid, AHAs remove the keratin to open and drain the pore, helping to make pores appear smaller and to improve the appearance of acne. Retinoids and benzoyl peroxide have achieved the same effect.

We know that breaking down keratin can help with acne, and ACV contains AHAs, so there is potential, but there are simply not functional studies to prove that.

If you are already using an anti-acne rinse or acne cream, and the treatment appears to irritate the body, causing dryness and peeling, and if you add ACV to your regimen, you may be removing the epidermis.

The object is accomplished by letting out all the moisture and everything inside— air pollutants, irritants, bacteria — in. Everyone is a bit different, and oily skin is likely to have a higher tolerance to apply more acidic products. There is a much lower threshold for sensitive, dry skin. There's no one-size-fits-all recommendation. Using ACV is less risky for teens with oily skin and acne because their skin is more resistant to irritation. The oil protects the skin's outer layer, and in a younger person, it comes back faster than an older adult with drier skin. Hair Benefits: In the medicine cabinet as well as in the kitchen cupboard, you may want to start stashing apple cider vinegar. This favorite ingredient can do more than just dress salads and make pickles — it's also a great all-in-one beauty product on a budget for you.

Apple cider vinegar can help you look beautiful from head to toe when used in your makeup routine. Hard soaps and shampoos often strip hair and skin of their natural oils, allowing you to feel dry all over. Apple cider vinegar acidity counteracts this cycle and in turn, improves the typical pH values of your skin and hair.

Make sure you get the right things. For the most beauty benefits, choose an organic brand of raw apple cider vinegar. Here are some useful tips on how to use apple cider vinegar to make your hair and skin look good.

For Hair

Apple cider vinegar removes product buildup, clumpy residue, and gunk from hair. Apple cider vinegar will revitalize your hair's body, making it moist and shiny when used daily in your natural hair care routine. The vinegar also acts by removing the skin cuticula, making it reflect light from it. In other words, this makes your hair super shiny!

Over the past few years, makeup advocates and medical experts have praised apple cider vinegar for its many health benefits, with many drinking apple cider vinegar to help clear their skin or even lose weight as part of their beauty routine. Like anything else, ACV may not be a miracle cure for any health-related issues, but helping you get bright, healthy hair can be an easy, economical workaround, whether you buy products such as apple cider vinegar shampoo or whipping a DIY hair rinse at home using ACV.

Apple Cider Vinegar for Optimal Health

Apple cider vinegar is much more than just an addition to your recipes. Due to its antibacterial, antifungal and antiviral properties, apple cider vinegar has been used to relieve various medical conditions by our ancestors.

Check out the list below to learn about the health benefits of ACV:

Diarrhea, intestinal spasms and other stomach issues – This vinegar has antibiotic properties which helps relieve tummy troubles caused by bacteria. Furthermore, apple cider vinegar contains pectin which helps soothe intestinal spasms.

Mix 2 tablespoons ACV in 1 glass of warm water and drink twice a day. This drink will relieve your symptoms quickly.

Sore throat – When your throat starts to feel itchy and sore, apple cider vinegar can help stop the infection. Mix ¼ cup of ACV in 1 glass of lukewarm water and gargle as often as needed. The acetic acid in this vinegar will relieve the itch. On the other hand, its antibacterial properties will prevent bacterial growth. You will feel relief as soon as you are done gargling with this mixture.

Foot odor and body odor – The acids in ACV helps balance the pH level of your skin. As a result, the odor-causing bacteria and germs that cause your underarm and feet smell are eliminated. Soak individual tissue papers, paper towels or baby wipes overnight in apple cider vinegar. Store in an air-tight container or zip lock and keep in the fridge for a day. Use it as needed. Although this vinegar has a strong acidic smell, it does go away when it dries.

Itch Relief – This all-around vinegar is also great for relieving itch caused by insect bites. It also provides great relief for jelly fish sting. Just apply ACV (Apple Cider Vinegar) directly on the affected area and feel relieved instantly.

Lower Cholesterol – In one study, the acetic acid found in apple cider vinegar caused a drop in the bad cholesterol level in lab rats. Another study also showed that apple cider vinegar helps reduce blood pressure in rats. Unfortunately, these results still need to be tested in humans. One Japanese study showed that people who consumed half an ounce of apple cider vinegar everyday has lower cholesterol level. This result still needs to be studied further.

Stuffy Nose – Apple cider vinegar contains potassium which helps thin mucus. It also contains acetic acid that prevents the growth of bacteria, therefore preventing nasal congestion. Mix 1 tablespoon of ACV in a glass of warm water and drink early in the morning and before sleeping to help drain your sinus.

Lower Blood Sugar Level – Drinking apple cider vinegar helps improve insulin sensitivity and lowers blood sugar response during meals. That being said, ACV is beneficial for people with diabetes or for those who are not diabetic but wants to keep their blood sugar levels to normal. Just drink 2 tablespoons of this multi-purpose vinegar before going to bed to reduce your blood sugar by up to 4%.

Weight Loss – The acetic acid found in ACV suppresses your appetite and increases your satiety. Therefore, it makes you feel fuller and lets you eat lesser. Research also suggests that ACV makes you eat lesser calories because it interferes with your body's digestion of starch, resulting to fewer calories entering your bloodstream.

Take 1 tablespoon of apple cider vinegar before each meal to help you reduce weight. You may also combine 3 parts ACV to 1 part olive oil and use it to massage your problem areas to help reduce your body fats.

Energy Drink – If you feel tired or weary or simply out of energy, give yourself a boost by adding 2 tablespoons of apple cider vinegar in a glass of water. You may add a tablespoon of honey for a little bit of sweetness. The enzymes and potassium found in ACV will boost your energy and take you to a higher gear.

Sunburn Relief – If your entire body is affected by sunburn, mix 1 cup of apple cider vinegar in your cool bath water and soak for 15 to 20 minutes. Pat your body dry and apply ACV directly on needed areas.

Headache – Vaporized ACV works wonders. Add 2 tablespoons of apple cider vinegar in a vaporizer or a pan with purified water. Heat the mixture until it boils. Remove from heat and place a towel over your head and lean on the pan of steaming ACV mixture. Breathe the steam vapors.

Yeast Infection – Add a cup of raw, undiluted apple cider vinegar in your warm bath. Soak in the warm bath mixture for 15 to 20 minutes. Do this during your morning bath and before going to bed at night.

External Itching – If you are experiencing itch due to allergic reactions, dry skin or imbalance in your body, simply dilute ¼ cup of ACV in 1 cup of water. Soak a cotton ball in the mixture and apply directly on the itch. Use as needed.

Leg Cramps and Swollen Muscles – Mix 2 tablespoons raw ACV in 1 cup of warm water and use it to massage the painful areas. The potassium in ACV will relieve your muscle spasm.

Hiccups – Hiccups can be very annoying and distracting. To get rid of hiccups, drink 1 to 2 tablespoons ACV. You'll be surprised at how fast your hiccups were relieved.

Urinary Tract Infection – Drink 2 tablespoons of ACV in the morning and in the evening. ACV will restore your body's natural pH balance. It will also prevent the growth of bacteria that causes UTI.

Dog Fleas – To fight off those pesky fleas from your dog, add 2 tablespoons of Apple cider vinegar in 1 liter of water and use it as the final rinse during your dog's bath. Your dog will be free from fleas and will have smoother, odor-free hair instantly.

Summary Conclusion

Apple cider vinegar is a wonderful elixir. Including it in your daily diet can be very easy. So welcome health, elegance, and strength with as little as a teaspoon of this incredible fluid a day into your life. There's no part of your body excluded from experiencing the amazing effects of apple cider vinegar, practically from the top to toe, inside and outside; if you use it daily, your body will enjoy something tasty.

The ACV is a product readily available that can be easily incorporated into meals. Large-scale work has shown its beneficial properties as a whole material, as well as the strengths of acetic acid and chlorogenic acid in the individual components. ACV can help control blood glucose and lipids, weight loss, and obesity, and can, therefore, be useful for treating type 2 diabetes. Although there is no work directly comparing acetic acid and ACV, ACV as a whole may be more active than acetic acid alone. Consumption of the' vinegar mom' can also improve beneficial effects relative to the lack of this element of ACV. It has been shown that the ACV production method alters the ACV components, which can, in turn, affect the beneficial qualities. To determine the extent of the influence of the production method, further research may be useful here. ACV use may help control type 2 diabetes.

There are NUMEROUS published studies done on ACV and it's weight loss effects, cleansing action and overall health benefits for people all over the world for a long time.

**Check out one of our other titles on Apple Cider Vinegar! Available on Amazon today! As always, order the Paperback version today
and get the Kindle version for FREE!**

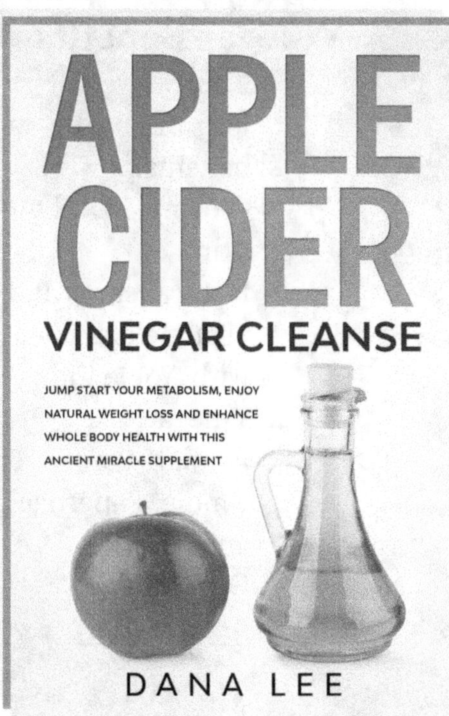

Apple Cider Vinegar Cleanse

- ✓ Jumpstart your metabolism
- ✓ Enjoy natural weightless
- ✓ Enhance whole body health with this ancient miracle supplement.
- ✓ Available on Kindle, Paperback and Audible.
- ✓ **Get Instant Access Here..**

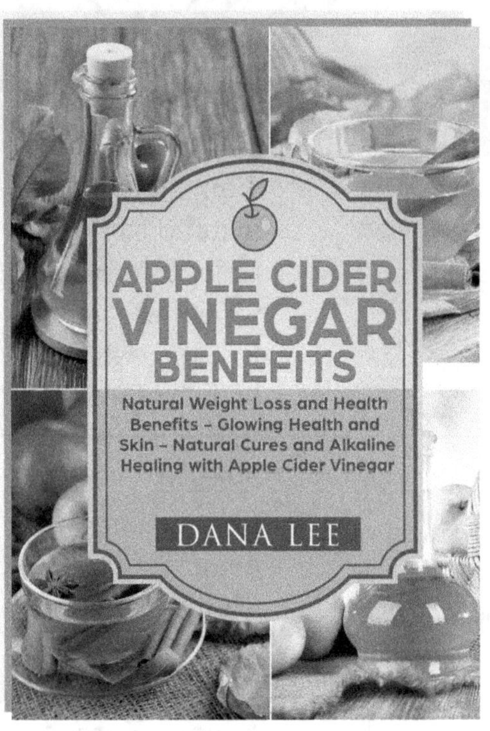

The Apple Cider Vinegar Benefits

- ✓ Natural weight loss and health benefits.
- ✓ Glowing healthy skin.
- ✓ Natural cures and alkaline healing with Apple Cider Vinegar!
- ✓ Available on Kindle, Paperback and Audible.
- ✓ **<u>Get Instant Access Here</u>**.